CHAIR PILATES FOR WOMEN OVER 40

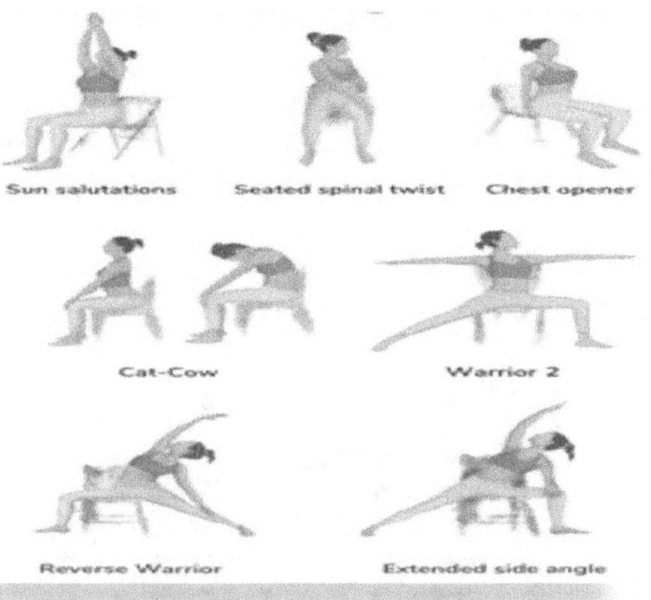

10 minutes daily exercise to ease back pain, strengthen your core, improve your balance, posture and prevent injury for beginners. (49 days body sculpting challenge and workout progress tracker)

CARLY EVELYN

SCAN TO GET MORE BOOKS BY THIS AUTHOR

IF YOU ARE STUCK, WHILE PRACTICING THE EXERCISE IN THIS GUIDE, YOU CAN REACH THE AUTHOR AT TRAINERCCARLY@GMAIL.COM FOR GUIDANCE

TABLE OF CONTENT

INTRODUCTION

In the quiet enclave of Willow Springs, a small town nestled between rolling hills and meandering streams, lived a woman named Olivia. She was known for her quiet determination and unyielding spirit. One day, as the golden rays of the morning sun painted the sky with hues of pink and orange, Olivia stumbled upon an old, dusty chair in the corner of her attic.

Curiosity sparkled in her eyes as she inspected the chair. Its wooden frame seemed to whisper tales of days gone by, but Olivia saw more than just a relic of the past. It was a canvas for transformation, an opportunity waiting to unfold. Inspired by a recent fitness revelation, she envisioned the chair as the perfect prop for her Pilates journey.

With newfound excitement, Olivia dusted off the chair and carried it into her living room. She cleared a space, creating a makeshift studio bathed in the soft glow of the morning light. As she settled onto the chair, she felt a surge of anticipation coursing through her veins.

With each controlled movement, Olivia began to unlock the potential within the chair. Its backrest became a support for her spine, the armrests a stabilizing force for her core. She flowed seamlessly from one exercise to the next, guided by the rhythm of her breath and the creaking of the aged chair.

It became an extension of her body, a partner in her pursuit of strength and flexibility.

Word of Olivia's unconventional Pilates sessions spread through the town like wildfire. Friends and neighbors gathered, intrigued by the transformation happening in Olivia's living room. The chair, once forgotten and relegated to the shadows, now took center stage as a symbol of empowerment and resilience.

As Olivia continued her daily practice, the effects were undeniable. Her posture improved, her muscles sculpted, and a radiant energy emanated from her. The chair, with its rustic charm, had become a beacon of inspiration for the community. People began to embrace the idea that transformation could emerge from the most unexpected places.

One day, as the sun dipped below the horizon, casting a warm glow over Willow Springs, Olivia stood tall beside the chair that had become her Pilates companion. A sense of accomplishment radiated from her, and the once-neglected chair stood as a testament to the power of determination and creativity.

In the heart of Willow Springs, Olivia's Pilates journey had not only transformed her physically but had also ignited a spark of possibility in the hearts of those who witnessed her remarkable metamorphosis. And so, in the quiet enclave, the chair stood as a silent witness to the extraordinary tale of a woman who found strength, grace, and resilience in the most unlikely of places.

STEP BY STEP GUIDE WITH PICTURE ILLUSTRATION

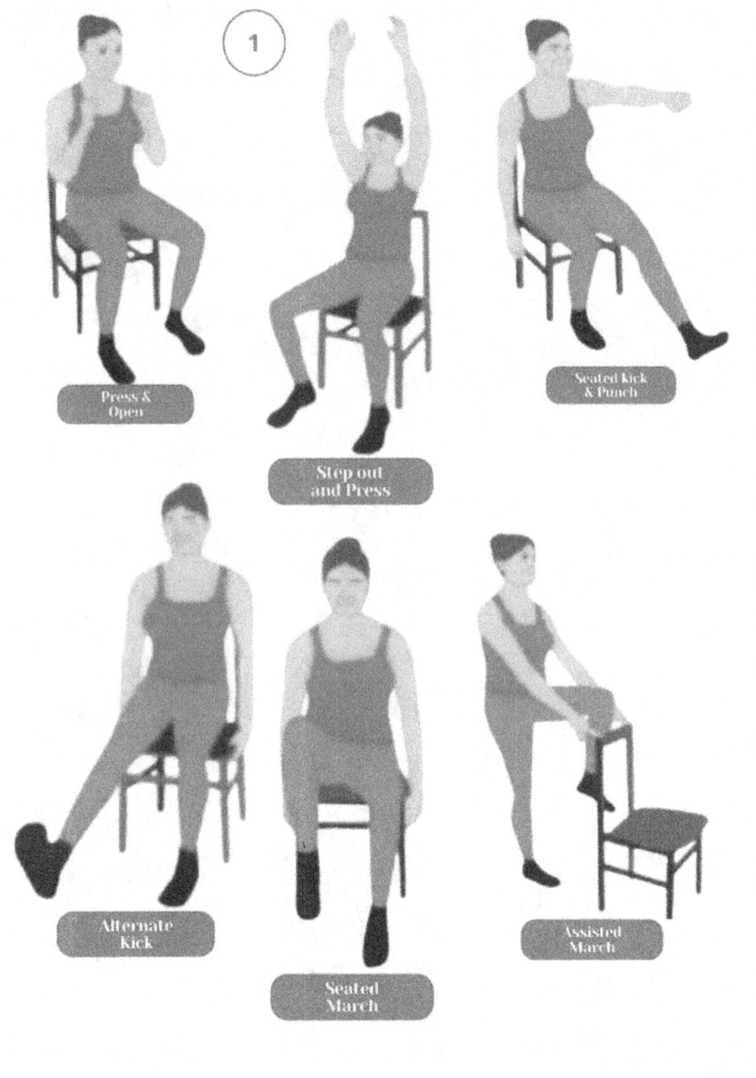

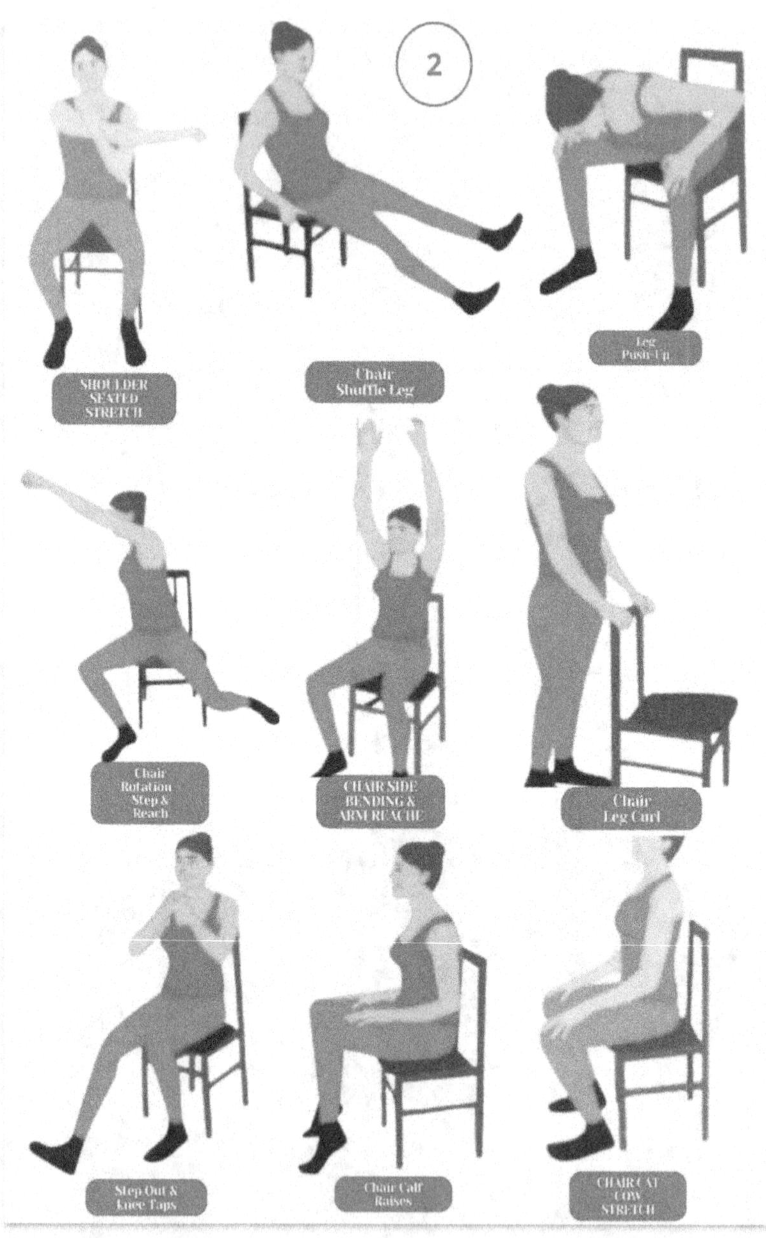

2
SHOULDER SEATED STRETCH
Chair Shuffle Leg
Leg Push-Up
Chair Rotation Step & Reach
CHAIR SIDE BENDING & ARM REACHE
Chair Leg Curl
Step-Out & Knee Taps
Chair Calf Raises
CHAIR CAT COW STRETCH

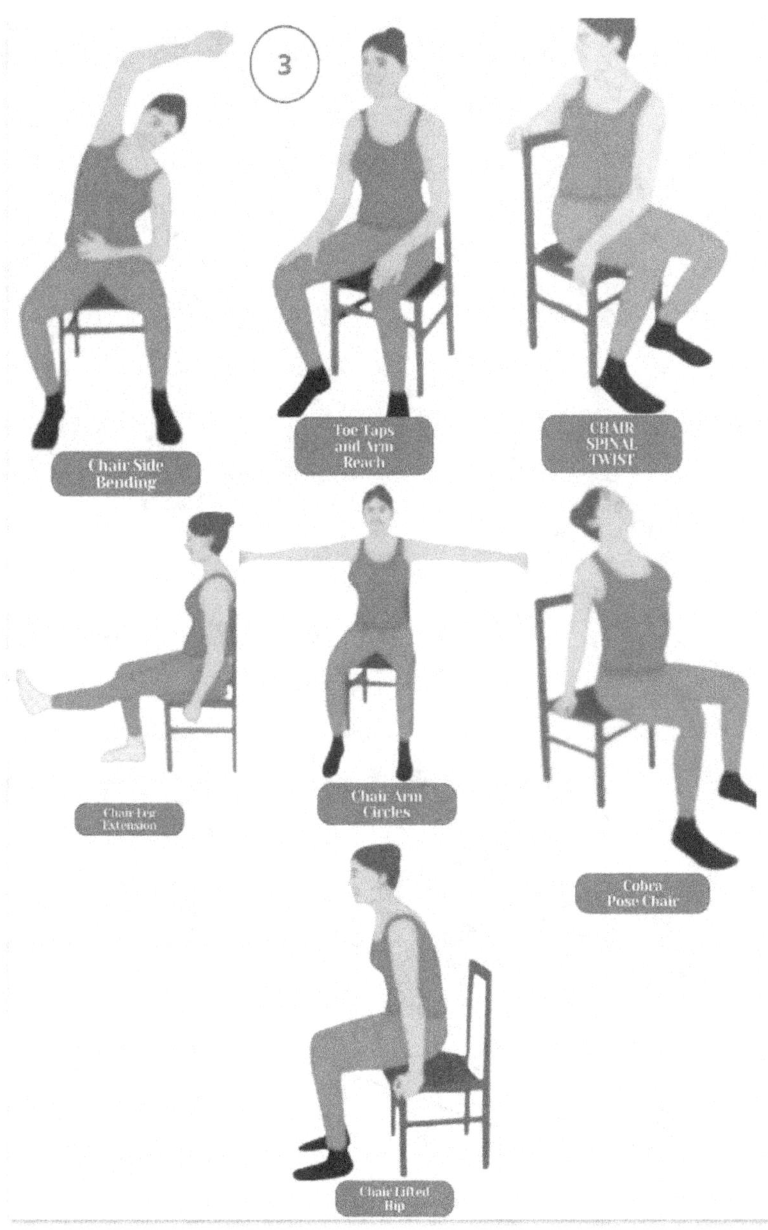
3
Chair Side
Bending
Toe Taps
and Arm
Reach
CHAIR
SPINAL
TWIST
Chair Leg
Extension
Chair Arm
Circles
Cobra
Pose Chair
Chair Lifted
Hip

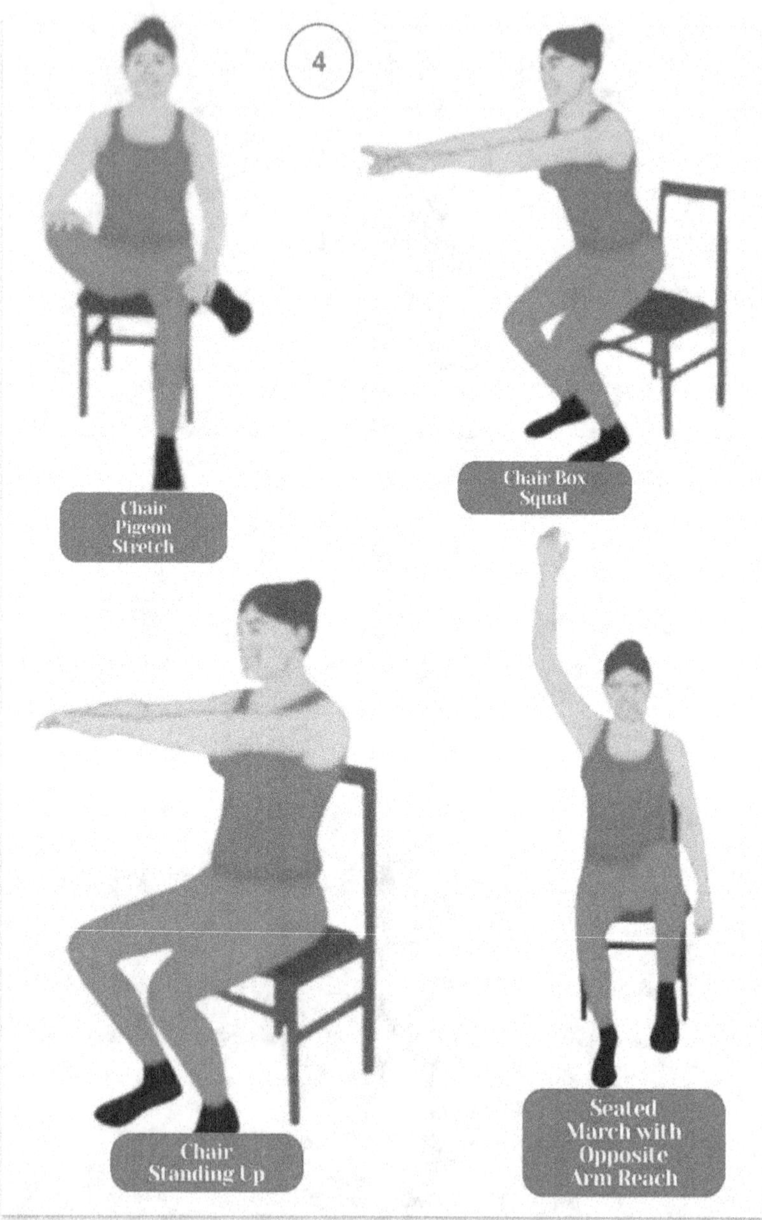
4
Chair
Pigeon
Stretch
Chair Box
Squat
Chair
Standing Up
Seated
March with
Opposite
Arm Reach

Chair Pilates presents a modified approach to the traditional Pilates method, integrating a chair as a versatile prop for a diverse range of exercises. Crafted to amplify strength, flexibility, and overall fitness, this innovative fitness routine may not feature precisely 40 exercises, but it delivers a varied set of examples accompanied by detailed step-by-step instructions. As with any new exercise regimen, it's crucial to seek guidance from a fitness professional or healthcare provider prior to commencement.

40 CHAIR PILATES EXERCISES TAILORED FOR WOMEN OVER 40.

1. Seated Arm Circles:
   - Assume a seated position on the chair with feet hip-width apart.
   - Extend your arms to shoulder height on each side.
   - Execute 10 forward arm circles followed by 10 in the reverse direction.

2. Seated Leg Lifts:
   - Sit on the chair's edge with a straight back.
   - Elevate one leg straight in front, lowering it without making contact with the floor.

- Repeat this sequence for both legs, completing 15 repetitions per leg.

3. Chair Squats:
   - Stand in front of the chair with feet hip-width apart.
   - Descend into a squat, ensuring knees remain over ankles.
   - Ascend back up, contracting the glutes. Perform 12 repetitions.

4. Seated Twist:
   - Sit tall and cross arms over the chest.
   - Rotate the torso to one side, then to the other.
   - Execute 15 reps for each side.

5. Single-Leg Circle:
   - Sit on the chair's edge, extending one leg straight.
   - Perform clockwise leg circles for 10 repetitions, then switch to counter-clockwise.

6. Chair Plank:
   - Position hands on the seat and extend feet backward.
   - Maintain a straight line from head to heels for 30 seconds.

7. Side Leg Lifts:
   - Sit sideways on the chair, supported by one hand.

- Elevate the upper leg and lower it without touching the lower leg.
   - Complete 15 reps for each side.

8. Chest Opener:
   - Sit tall, clasping hands behind the back.
   - Slightly lift arms, opening the chest.

9. Standing Oblique Crunch:
   - Stand with hands behind the head.
   - Draw one knee towards the same-side elbow.

10. Chair Dip:
   - Sit on the chair's edge, gripping the seat with hands.
   - Lower and lift the body by bending the elbows.

11. Seated Bicycle Crunch:
   - Sit tall, raising feet off the ground.
   - Rotate the torso, bringing one knee towards the chest.

12. Chair Bridge:
   - Sit on the chair's edge with hands on the sides.
   - Elevate hips towards the ceiling, engaging glutes.

13. Side Plank on Chair:
   - Place one hand on the seat, lifting hips.
   - Hold for 20 seconds on each side.

14. Chair Lunges:

- Stand facing away from the chair.
- Step one foot back into a lunge position.

15. Armchair Push-Ups:

- Position hands on the chair's arms.
- Lower and lift the body by bending the elbows.

16. Chair Mountain Climbers:

- Place hands on the seat, arms fully extended.
- Bring one knee towards the chest, then alternate quickly.

17. Seated Side Stretch:

- Sit tall, extending one arm overhead.
- Incline the torso to one side, creating a stretch along the torso.

18. Knee Extensions:

- Sit tall, extending one leg straight.
- Flex and point the foot, engaging the thigh muscles.

19. Seated Scissors:

- Sit on the chair's edge, lifting both legs off the ground.
- Open and close legs in a scissor-like motion.

20. Chair Forward Bend:

- Sit tall, hinge at the hips, reaching towards the floor.

- Hold for 20 seconds, feeling the hamstring stretch.

21. Toe Taps:
- Sit on the chair's edge, lifting both feet off the ground.
- Alternately tap toes on the floor.

22. Seated Back Extension:
- Sit tall, clasping hands behind the back.
- Lift arms slightly, arching the back.

23. Chair Side Crunch:
- Sit tall, placing one hand on the seat.
- Elevate the leg on the same side towards the elbow.

24. Lateral Leg Raises:
- Stand beside the chair, lifting one leg to the side.
- Lower and lift for 15 reps, then switch sides.

25. Chair Calf Raises:
- Stand behind the chair, rising onto tiptoes.
- Lower heels back down, repeating for 20 reps.

26. Seated Knee Circles:
- Sit tall, lifting one knee and circling it in one direction.
- Change directions after 10 reps, then switch legs.

27. Chair Reverse Plank:
   - Sit on the chair's edge, placing hands on the seat.
   - Elevate hips towards the ceiling, facing forward.

28. Seated Mermaid Stretch:
   - Sit with legs to one side, placing one hand on the seat.
   - Extend the opposite arm overhead, creating a side stretch.

29. Leg Pull Front:
   - Sit tall, lifting hips off the chair.
   - Extend one leg forward, holding for a few seconds before switching.

30. Chair Oblique Twist:
   - Sit tall, holding the sides of the chair.
   - Twist the torso to one side, then the other.

31. Seated High Knees:
   - Sit tall, rapidly lifting knees towards the chest.

32. Chair Side Plank with Leg Lift:
   - Place one hand on the seat, lifting hips.
   - Elevate the top leg, engaging the side muscles.

33. Seated Side Leg Twist:
   - Sit tall, lifting both legs off the ground.
   - Twist the torso to one side, then the other.

34. Chair Superman:
   - Sit on the chair's edge, extending arms forward and lifting legs.
   - Hold for 10 seconds, engaging the core and lower back.

35. Seated Hip Flexor Stretch:
   - Sit tall, crossing one ankle over the opposite knee.
   - Gently press down on the lifted knee.

36. Chair Side Lunges:
   - Stand beside the chair, stepping one leg out to the side.
   - Bend the knee and push hips back.

37. Seated Boat Pose:
   - Sit tall, lifting legs off the ground, balancing on the sit bones.

38. Chair Triceps Kickbacks:
   - Sit tall, holding a weight in one hand.
   - Extend the arm straight back, engaging the triceps.

39. Seated Figure 4 Stretch:
   - Sit tall, crossing one ankle over the opposite knee.
   - Gently press down on the lifted knee.

40. Chair Burpees:

- Stand, placing hands on the seat, and jump feet back into a plank.

- Jump back in and stand up, repeating for 15 reps.

These chair Pilates exercises deliver a comprehensive workout, targeting diverse muscle groups. Ensure consistent form and intensity adjustments based on your fitness level, gradually progressing as you advance.

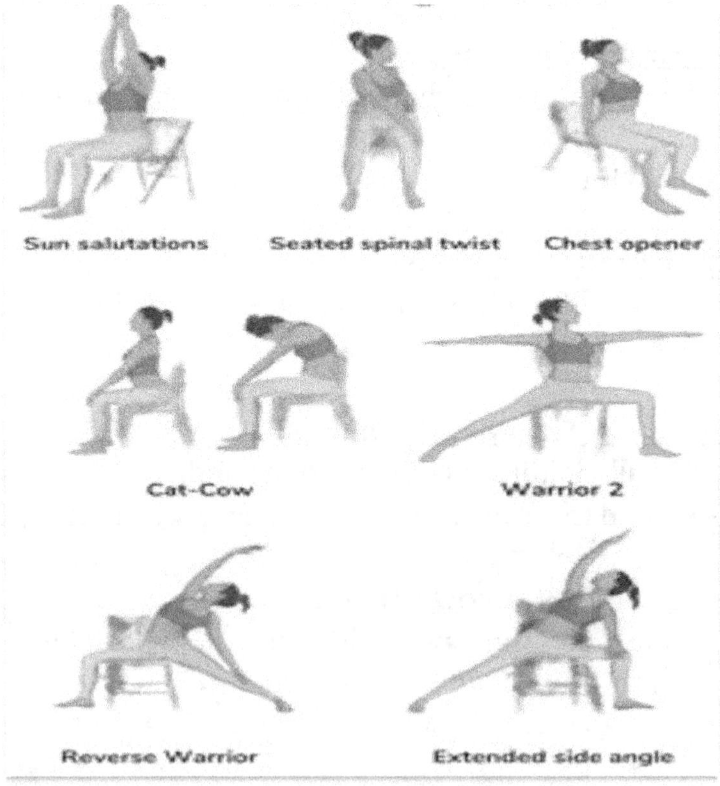

1. "Infuse strength into your body and mind with every Pilates motion; let the chair become your throne of empowerment."

2. "Within the fitness domain, the chair transforms into your unspoken companion, aiding your voyage towards a more robust and healthier self."

3. "Whether seated or upright, envision the chair as your canvas for metamorphosis. Craft an image of fortitude and resilience."

4. "Experience the potency of your core with each lift and twist. The chair transcends its role as a mere seat; it evolves into a vessel of transformation."

5. "In the realm of Pilates, consider the chair your steadfast ally — a firm base for your journey toward achieving greatness."

6. "Never underestimate the chair; it serves a purpose beyond sitting. It acts as a tool for

chiseling a version of yourself that exudes
strength and confidence."

7. "Though the chair may appear immobile,
each Pilates movement propels you towards a
more vibrant and energetic rendition of
yourself."

8. "Embrace the chair as your fitness
companion, allowing it to steer you towards
new heights of strength and flexibility."

9. "Metamorphose your chair into a throne of
well-being. Every Pilates session becomes a
coronation, affirming your commitment to
self-care."

10. "Whether seated or soaring, the chair
adjusts to your tempo. Let it orchestrate the
melody of your Pilates symphony."

11. "While you sit, rise, and move, bear in
mind: the chair is your fitness chariot,
propelling you toward a life that is healthier
and more vibrant."

12. "Regard the chair as your Pilates
confidant, aiding you in sculpting the
masterpiece that is your body."

13. "Shape your strength on the chair's throne. Each movement acts as a stroke, contributing to the masterpiece of your fitness journey."

14. "Participating in Pilates on a chair is more than an exercise; it's a pledge to your well-being. Each movement is a stride toward a healthier version of yourself."

15. "Sense the grace in every seated stretch and the force in every lift. The chair serves as your gateway to a body that is both balanced and robust."

16. "Though your fitness journey commences on the chair, it extends beyond. It acts as a launchpad to a life characterized by strength, balance, and vitality."

17. "The strength derived from sitting lays the foundation for standing resilience. Allow the chair to be your anchor as you navigate the undulating waves of your Pilates practice."

18. "Within the Pilates domain, the chair acts as your guide, pointing you toward a destination characterized by health, vitality, and self-discovery."

19. "Your Pilates expedition on the chair is not merely an exercise; it's a jubilation of the incredible strength and resilience inherent within you."

20. "The chair transcends its identity as a piece of furniture; it symbolizes your dedication to a life that is fit and vibrant."

21. "Pilates on a chair becomes a dance of strength and flexibility. Let each movement choreograph a narrative of empowerment."

22. "Whether sitting tall or standing strong, the chair acts as the bridge between the two. Embrace it, allowing your strength to unfurl."

23. "As you sit and move, don't forget: the chair doesn't merely support your body; it elevates your spirit."

24. "While on the chair, you're not just exercising; you're crafting a version of yourself that emanates strength, balance, and grace."

25. "Whether seated or soaring, you're in command. The chair becomes your

instrument; allow it to compose the melody of your strength."

26. "Each Pilates move on the chair propels you toward a life that is healthier and more vibrant. Embrace the journey, savoring each mindful movement."

27. "Consider the chair your personal gym, where every exercise is an opportunity to sculpt your body and enhance your well-being."

28. "The foundational strength derived from sitting serves as the anchor for standing resilience. Allow the chair to guide you through the undulating waves of your Pilates practice."

29. "The chair isn't merely a support; it propels you toward strength, resilience, and a healthier version of yourself. Whether seated or standing, let every movement testify to your commitment."

30. "While on the chair, you're not just exercising; you're sculpting a version of yourself that radiates strength, balance, and

grace. Embrace the journey, one mindful movement at a time."

BONUS

air
squats
burpees
bicycle
crunches
kick backs
(left)
jump
squats
kick backs
(right)
push ups
side plank
(left)
mountain
climbers
side plank
(right)
triceps
push ups
high knee
run
sumo
squats
triceps
dips
jumping
jacks

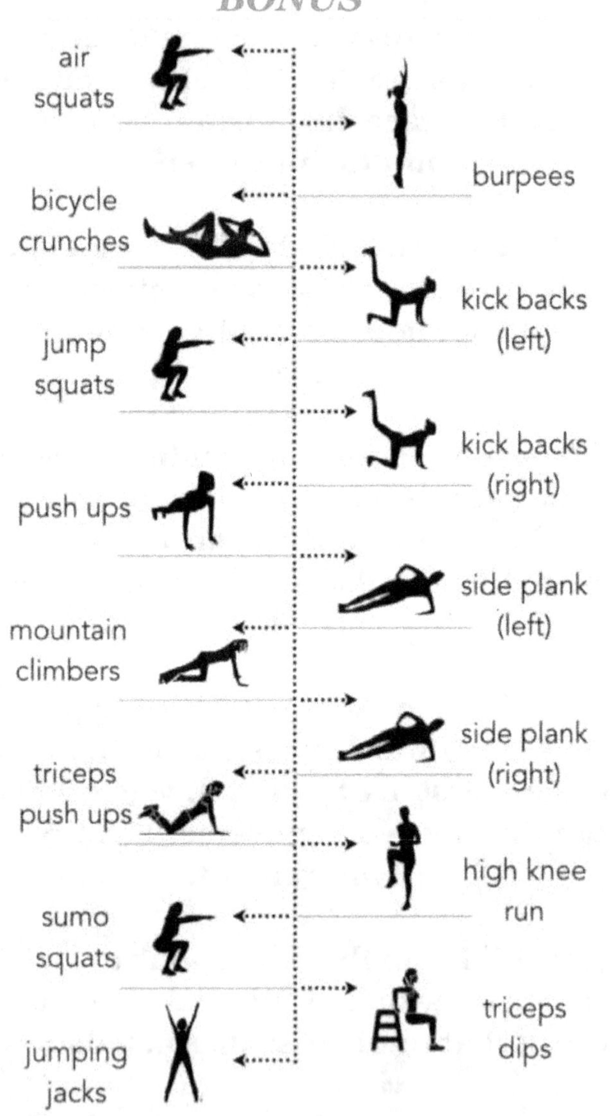

CONCLUSION

In the closing pages of this chair Pilates exercises guide for women, we embark on a journey that extends beyond the physical movements on a simple piece of furniture. What began as a collection of exercises evolves into a narrative of empowerment, resilience, and self-discovery.

As you turn the last page, envision the chair not merely as an object but as a catalyst for transformation. It symbolizes your commitment to well-being, your dedication to sculpting strength, and your canvas for creating a healthier, more vibrant you. Each exercise is a brushstroke, contributing to the masterpiece of your fitness journey.

In the quiet moments of reflection after completing these exercises, may you recognize the power within yourself—the power to rise, transform, and embrace a life of balance, grace, and strength. The chair becomes more than just a tool; it becomes a companion in your quest for a healthier, more empowered existence.

This guide is not just about Pilates on a chair; it's about redefining what is possible for your body, mind, and spirit. As you step off the chair and into the world, carry with you the lessons learned, the strength gained, and the resilience cultivated. Your fitness journey is a continuous story, and this book is but one chapter—a chapter that inspires you to keep turning the pages, exploring new movements, and embracing the limitless possibilities that lie ahead.

May the chair Pilates exercises within these pages be the starting point for a life where every movement is intentional, every breath is powerful, and every day is a celebration of your journey towards optimal well-being. Here's to the empowered, resilient, and vibrant woman you are becoming, one chair Pilates exercise at a time.

THANK YOU!!!!
IF YOU INSPIRED AND FIND THE
INFORMATION IN THIS BOOK
HELPFUL, DON'T FORGET TO
GIVE THIS BOOK A REVIEW ON
AMAZON. YOUR FEEDBACKS
WILL GO A LONG WAY THANKS

CHAIR PILATES WORKOUT PROGRESS TRACKER

Weekly Workout Progress Tracker

WEEK OF THE MONTH: _______________

TYPE OF EXERCISE:	MUSCLE GROUP:	REPS:	S M T W T F S
_____________	_____________	_______	○○○○○○○
_____________	_____________	_______	○○○○○○○
_____________	_____________	_______	○○○○○○○
_____________	_____________	_______	○○○○○○○
_____________	_____________	_______	○○○○○○○
_____________	_____________	_______	○○○○○○○
_____________	_____________	_______	○○○○○○○

WHAT I LIKED ABOUT THIS WORKOUT:

WHAT I WILL CHANGE FOR NEXT WEEK:

WHAT I NOTICED WEEKLY ON MY BODY

WATER:

S M T W T F S
○○○○○○○

MEAL PLAN:

S M T W T F S
○○○○○○○

Weekly Workout Progress Tracker

WEEK OF THE MONTH: _______________

TYPE OF EXERCISE:	MUSCLE GROUP:	REPS:	S M T W T F S
			○○○○○○○
TYPE OF EXERCISE:	MUSCLE GROUP:	REPS:	S M T W T F S
			○○○○○○○
TYPE OF EXERCISE:	MUSCLE GROUP:	REPS:	S M T W T F S
			○○○○○○○
TYPE OF EXERCISE:	MUSCLE GROUP:	REPS:	S M T W T F S
			○○○○○○○
TYPE OF EXERCISE:	MUSCLE GROUP:	REPS:	S M T W T F S
			○○○○○○○
TYPE OF EXERCISE:	MUSCLE GROUP:	REPS:	S M T W T F S
			○○○○○○○
TYPE OF EXERCISE:	MUSCLE GROUP:	REPS:	S M T W T F S
			○○○○○○○

WHAT I LIKED ABOUT THIS WORKOUT:

WHAT I WILL CHANGE FOR NEXT WEEK:

WHAT I NOTICED WEEKLY ON MY BODY

WATER:

S M T W T F S
○○○○○○○

MEAL PLAN:

S M T W T F S
○○○○○○○

Weekly Workout Progress Tracker

WEEK OF THE MONTH: _______________

TYPE OF EXERCISE:	MUSCLE GROUP:	REPS:	S M T W T F S
_____________	_____________	_______	○○○○○○○
TYPE OF EXERCISE:	MUSCLE GROUP:	REPS:	S M T W T F S
_____________	_____________	_______	○○○○○○○
TYPE OF EXERCISE:	MUSCLE GROUP:	REPS:	S M T W T F S
_____________	_____________	_______	○○○○○○○
TYPE OF EXERCISE:	MUSCLE GROUP:	REPS:	S M T W T F S
_____________	_____________	_______	○○○○○○○
TYPE OF EXERCISE:	MUSCLE GROUP:	REPS:	S M T W T F S
_____________	_____________	_______	○○○○○○○
TYPE OF EXERCISE:	MUSCLE GROUP:	REPS:	S M T W T F S
_____________	_____________	_______	○○○○○○○
TYPE OF EXERCISE:	MUSCLE GROUP:	REPS:	S M T W T F S
_____________	_____________	_______	○○○○○○○

WHAT I LIKED ABOUT THIS WORKOUT:

WHAT I WILL CHANGE FOR NEXT WEEK:

WHAT I NOTICED WEEKLY ON MY BODY

WATER:

S M T W T F S

○○○○○○○

MEAL PLAN:

S M T W T F S

○○○○○○○

Weekly Workout Progress Tracker

WEEK OF THE MONTH: _______________

TYPE OF EXERCISE:	MUSCLE GROUP:	REPS:	S M T W T F S
_______________	_______________	_______	○○○○○○○
TYPE OF EXERCISE:	MUSCLE GROUP:	REPS:	S M T W T F S
_______________	_______________	_______	○○○○○○○
TYPE OF EXERCISE:	MUSCLE GROUP:	REPS:	S M T W T F S
_______________	_______________	_______	○○○○○○○
TYPE OF EXERCISE:	MUSCLE GROUP:	REPS:	S M T W T F S
_______________	_______________	_______	○○○○○○○
TYPE OF EXERCISE:	MUSCLE GROUP:	REPS:	S M T W T F S
_______________	_______________	_______	○○○○○○○
TYPE OF EXERCISE:	MUSCLE GROUP:	REPS:	S M T W T F S
_______________	_______________	_______	○○○○○○○
TYPE OF EXERCISE:	MUSCLE GROUP:	REPS:	S M T W T F S
_______________	_______________	_______	○○○○○○○

WHAT I LIKED ABOUT THIS WORKOUT:

WHAT I WILL CHANGE FOR NEXT WEEK:

WHAT I NOTICED WEEKLY ON MY BODY

WATER:

S M T W T F S

○○○○○○○

MEAL PLAN:

S M T W T F S

○○○○○○○

Weekly Workout Progress Tracker

WEEK OF THE MONTH: _______________

TYPE OF EXERCISE:	MUSCLE GROUP:	REPS:	S M T W T F S
_______________	_______________	_______	○○○○○○○
TYPE OF EXERCISE:	MUSCLE GROUP:	REPS:	S M T W T F S
_______________	_______________	_______	○○○○○○○
TYPE OF EXERCISE:	MUSCLE GROUP:	REPS:	S M T W T F S
_______________	_______________	_______	○○○○○○○
TYPE OF EXERCISE:	MUSCLE GROUP:	REPS:	S M T W T F S
_______________	_______________	_______	○○○○○○○
TYPE OF EXERCISE:	MUSCLE GROUP:	REPS:	S M T W T F S
_______________	_______________	_______	○○○○○○○
TYPE OF EXERCISE:	MUSCLE GROUP:	REPS:	S M T W T F S
_______________	_______________	_______	○○○○○○○
TYPE OF EXERCISE:	MUSCLE GROUP:	REPS:	S M T W T F S
_______________	_______________	_______	○○○○○○○

WHAT I LIKED ABOUT THIS WORKOUT:

WHAT I WILL CHANGE FOR NEXT WEEK:

WHAT I NOTICED WEEKLY ON MY BODY

<u>WATER:</u>

S M T W T F S

○○○○○○○

<u>MEAL PLAN:</u>

S M T W T F S

○○○○○○○

Weekly Workout Progress Tracker

WEEK OF THE MONTH: _________________

TYPE OF EXERCISE:	MUSCLE GROUP:	REPS:	S M T W T F S
_____________	_____________	_______	O O O O O O O
TYPE OF EXERCISE:	MUSCLE GROUP:	REPS:	S M T W T F S
_____________	_____________	_______	O O O O O O O
TYPE OF EXERCISE:	MUSCLE GROUP:	REPS:	S M T W T F S
_____________	_____________	_______	O O O O O O O
TYPE OF EXERCISE:	MUSCLE GROUP:	REPS:	S M T W T F S
_____________	_____________	_______	O O O O O O O
TYPE OF EXERCISE:	MUSCLE GROUP:	REPS:	S M T W T F S
_____________	_____________	_______	O O O O O O O
TYPE OF EXERCISE:	MUSCLE GROUP:	REPS:	S M T W T F S
_____________	_____________	_______	O O O O O O O
TYPE OF EXERCISE:	MUSCLE GROUP:	REPS:	S M T W T F S
_____________	_____________	_______	O O O O O O O

WHAT I LIKED ABOUT THIS WORKOUT:

WATER:

S M T W T F S

O O O O O O O

WHAT I WILL CHANGE FOR NEXT WEEK:

WHAT I NOTICED WEEKLY ON MY BODY

MEAL PLAN:

S M T W T F S

O O O O O O O

Weekly Workout Progress Tracker

WEEK OF THE MONTH: _______________

TYPE OF EXERCISE:	MUSCLE GROUP:	REPS:	S M T W T F S
			○ ○ ○ ○ ○ ○ ○

TYPE OF EXERCISE:	MUSCLE GROUP:	REPS:	S M T W T F S
			○ ○ ○ ○ ○ ○ ○

TYPE OF EXERCISE:	MUSCLE GROUP:	REPS:	S M T W T F S
			○ ○ ○ ○ ○ ○ ○

TYPE OF EXERCISE:	MUSCLE GROUP:	REPS:	S M T W T F S
			○ ○ ○ ○ ○ ○ ○

TYPE OF EXERCISE:	MUSCLE GROUP:	REPS:	S M T W T F S
			○ ○ ○ ○ ○ ○ ○

TYPE OF EXERCISE:	MUSCLE GROUP:	REPS:	S M T W T F S
			○ ○ ○ ○ ○ ○ ○

TYPE OF EXERCISE:	MUSCLE GROUP:	REPS:	S M T W T F S
			○ ○ ○ ○ ○ ○ ○

WHAT I LIKED ABOUT THIS WORKOUT:

WHAT I WILL CHANGE FOR NEXT WEEK:

WHAT I NOTICED WEEKLY ON MY BODY

WATER:

S M T W T F S

○ ○ ○ ○ ○ ○ ○

MEAL PLAN:

S M T W T F S

○ ○ ○ ○ ○ ○ ○

Weekly Workout Progress Tracker

WEEK OF THE MONTH: _______________

TYPE OF EXERCISE:	MUSCLE GROUP:	REPS:	S M T W T F S
_______________	_______________	_______	○○○○○○○
TYPE OF EXERCISE:	MUSCLE GROUP:	REPS:	S M T W T F S
_______________	_______________	_______	○○○○○○○
TYPE OF EXERCISE:	MUSCLE GROUP:	REPS:	S M T W T F S
_______________	_______________	_______	○○○○○○○
TYPE OF EXERCISE:	MUSCLE GROUP:	REPS:	S M T W T F S
_______________	_______________	_______	○○○○○○○
TYPE OF EXERCISE:	MUSCLE GROUP:	REPS:	S M T W T F S
_______________	_______________	_______	○○○○○○○
TYPE OF EXERCISE:	MUSCLE GROUP:	REPS:	S M T W T F S
_______________	_______________	_______	○○○○○○○
TYPE OF EXERCISE:	MUSCLE GROUP:	REPS:	S M T W T F S
_______________	_______________	_______	○○○○○○○

WHAT I LIKED ABOUT THIS WORKOUT:

WATER:

S M T W T F S
○○○○○○○

WHAT I WILL CHANGE FOR NEXT WEEK:

WHAT I NOTICED WEEKLY ON MY BODY

MEAL PLAN:

S M T W T F S
○○○○○○○

Weekly Workout
Progress Tracker
WEEK OF THE MONTH: _______________

TYPE OF EXERCISE:	MUSCLE GROUP:	REPS:	S M T W T F S
			O O O O O O O
TYPE OF EXERCISE:	MUSCLE GROUP:	REPS:	S M T W T F S
			O O O O O O O
TYPE OF EXERCISE:	MUSCLE GROUP:	REPS:	S M T W T F S
			O O O O O O O
TYPE OF EXERCISE:	MUSCLE GROUP:	REPS:	S M T W T F S
			O O O O O O O
TYPE OF EXERCISE:	MUSCLE GROUP:	REPS:	S M T W T F S
			O O O O O O O
TYPE OF EXERCISE:	MUSCLE GROUP:	REPS:	S M T W T F S
			O O O O O O O
TYPE OF EXERCISE:	MUSCLE GROUP:	REPS:	S M T W T F S
			O O O O O O O

WHAT I LIKED ABOUT THIS WORKOUT:

WATER:

S M T W T F S

O O O O O O O

WHAT I WILL CHANGE FOR NEXT WEEK:

WHAT I NOTICED WEEKLY ON MY BODY

MEAL PLAN:

S M T W T F S

O O O O O O O

Weekly Workout Progress Tracker

WEEK OF THE MONTH: _______________

TYPE OF EXERCISE:	MUSCLE GROUP:	REPS:	S M T W T F S
_______________	_______________	_______	○○○○○○○
TYPE OF EXERCISE:	MUSCLE GROUP:	REPS:	S M T W T F S
_______________	_______________	_______	○○○○○○○
TYPE OF EXERCISE:	MUSCLE GROUP:	REPS:	S M T W T F S
_______________	_______________	_______	○○○○○○○
TYPE OF EXERCISE:	MUSCLE GROUP:	REPS:	S M T W T F S
_______________	_______________	_______	○○○○○○○
TYPE OF EXERCISE:	MUSCLE GROUP:	REPS:	S M T W T F S
_______________	_______________	_______	○○○○○○○
TYPE OF EXERCISE:	MUSCLE GROUP:	REPS:	S M T W T F S
_______________	_______________	_______	○○○○○○○
TYPE OF EXERCISE:	MUSCLE GROUP:	REPS:	S M T W T F S
_______________	_______________	_______	○○○○○○○

WHAT I LIKED ABOUT THIS WORKOUT:

WATER:

S M T W T F S

○○○○○○○

WHAT I WILL CHANGE FOR NEXT WEEK:

WHAT I NOTICED WEEKLY ON MY BODY

MEAL PLAN:

S M T W T F S

○○○○○○○

Weekly Workout Progress Tracker

WEEK OF THE MONTH: ______________

TYPE OF EXERCISE:	MUSCLE GROUP:	REPS:	S M T W T F S
			○○○○○○○
TYPE OF EXERCISE:	MUSCLE GROUP:	REPS:	S M T W T F S
			○○○○○○○
TYPE OF EXERCISE:	MUSCLE GROUP:	REPS:	S M T W T F S
			○○○○○○○
TYPE OF EXERCISE:	MUSCLE GROUP:	REPS:	S M T W T F S
			○○○○○○○
TYPE OF EXERCISE:	MUSCLE GROUP:	REPS:	S M T W T F S
			○○○○○○○
TYPE OF EXERCISE:	MUSCLE GROUP:	REPS:	S M T W T F S
			○○○○○○○
TYPE OF EXERCISE:	MUSCLE GROUP:	REPS:	S M T W T F S
			○○○○○○○

WHAT I LIKED ABOUT THIS WORKOUT:

WHAT I WILL CHANGE FOR NEXT WEEK:

WHAT I NOTICED WEEKLY ON MY BODY

WATER:

S M T W T F S
○○○○○○○

MEAL PLAN:

S M T W T F S
○○○○○○○

Weekly Workout Progress Tracker

WEEK OF THE MONTH: _______________

TYPE OF EXERCISE:	MUSCLE GROUP:	REPS:	S M T W T F S
_______________	_______________	_______	○○○○○○○
TYPE OF EXERCISE:	MUSCLE GROUP:	REPS:	S M T W T F S
_______________	_______________	_______	○○○○○○○
TYPE OF EXERCISE:	MUSCLE GROUP:	REPS:	S M T W T F S
_______________	_______________	_______	○○○○○○○
TYPE OF EXERCISE:	MUSCLE GROUP:	REPS:	S M T W T F S
_______________	_______________	_______	○○○○○○○
TYPE OF EXERCISE:	MUSCLE GROUP:	REPS:	S M T W T F S
_______________	_______________	_______	○○○○○○○
TYPE OF EXERCISE:	MUSCLE GROUP:	REPS:	S M T W T F S
_______________	_______________	_______	○○○○○○○
TYPE OF EXERCISE:	MUSCLE GROUP:	REPS:	S M T W T F S
_______________	_______________	_______	○○○○○○○

WHAT I LIKED ABOUT THIS WORKOUT:

WATER:

S M T W T F S
○○○○○○○

WHAT I WILL CHANGE FOR NEXT WEEK:

WHAT I NOTICED WEEKLY ON MY BODY

MEAL PLAN:

S M T W T F S
○○○○○○○

Weekly Workout Progress Tracker

WEEK OF THE MONTH: _______________

TYPE OF EXERCISE:	MUSCLE GROUP:	REPS:	S M T W T F S
			○○○○○○○
TYPE OF EXERCISE:	MUSCLE GROUP:	REPS:	S M T W T F S
			○○○○○○○
TYPE OF EXERCISE:	MUSCLE GROUP:	REPS:	S M T W T F S
			○○○○○○○
TYPE OF EXERCISE:	MUSCLE GROUP:	REPS:	S M T W T F S
			○○○○○○○
TYPE OF EXERCISE:	MUSCLE GROUP:	REPS:	S M T W T F S
			○○○○○○○
TYPE OF EXERCISE:	MUSCLE GROUP:	REPS:	S M T W T F S
			○○○○○○○
TYPE OF EXERCISE:	MUSCLE GROUP:	REPS:	S M T W T F S
			○○○○○○○

WHAT I LIKED ABOUT THIS WORKOUT:

WHAT I WILL CHANGE FOR NEXT WEEK:

WHAT I NOTICED WEEKLY ON MY BODY

WATER:

S M T W T F S

○○○○○○○

MEAL PLAN:

S M T W T F S

○○○○○○○

Weekly Workout Progress Tracker

WEEK OF THE MONTH: ___________________

TYPE OF EXERCISE:	MUSCLE GROUP:	REPS:	S M T W T F S
_______________	_____________	______	○○○○○○○
TYPE OF EXERCISE:	MUSCLE GROUP:	REPS:	S M T W T F S
_______________	_____________	______	○○○○○○○
TYPE OF EXERCISE:	MUSCLE GROUP:	REPS:	S M T W T F S
_______________	_____________	______	○○○○○○○
TYPE OF EXERCISE:	MUSCLE GROUP:	REPS:	S M T W T F S
_______________	_____________	______	○○○○○○○
TYPE OF EXERCISE:	MUSCLE GROUP:	REPS:	S M T W T F S
_______________	_____________	______	○○○○○○○
TYPE OF EXERCISE:	MUSCLE GROUP:	REPS:	S M T W T F S
_______________	_____________	______	○○○○○○○
TYPE OF EXERCISE:	MUSCLE GROUP:	REPS:	S M T W T F S
_______________	_____________	______	○○○○○○○

WHAT I LIKED ABOUT THIS WORKOUT:

WHAT I WILL CHANGE FOR NEXT WEEK:

WHAT I NOTICED WEEKLY ON MY BODY

WATER:

S M T W T F S

○○○○○○○

MEAL PLAN:

S M T W T F S

○○○○○○○

www.ingramcontent.com/pod-product-compliance
Lightning Source LLC
Chambersburg PA
CBHW060855260726
48661CB00008B/3278